DYING TO KNOW

Straight Talk about Death and Dying

ISBN 10: 0-9789573-0-X
ISBN 13: 978-0-9789573-0-8

Nothing in life is to be feared.
It is only to be understood.
—Marie Curie

Dedication

In honor of and in gratitude to all my patients and their families, who shared their journeys and taught me about living well and dying well.

Acknowledgements

Whether through the encouragement and support that friend-
ship provides or by sharing stories and providing feedback on
the drafts, the following have contributed to making this book a
reality. I will be forever grateful.

Ed Beggy
David Christensen
Bayla Cohen
Carol Cooper Garey
Ardie DelForge
Eric Gaines
Justin Gaines
Todd Gaines
Gary Malkin
Jane Martin
Elaine Rousseau
Ann Orlov Rubinow
Michael Ryan
Mary Jo Spring
Joan Stempel
Ed Weiser
Richard Weiser

Table of Contents

Preface

The art of living well and dying well are one.
—Epicurus

There are no better teachers of the dying process than the patients and families who are experiencing it. For over thirty years, I have been privileged to be their student by bearing witness to and playing a role in this sacred process. What a gift that people have shared their lives' ends and their insights, revealing the full spectrum of this amazing experience, from tragedies to blessings, pain to comfort, and fear to peace. One of their stated keys to meeting the challenges was receiving honest information delivered simply and compassionately so they knew what to expect and how to confront it.

The purpose of this book is to share what these amazing teachers have taught me about dying. This book is for you, the person given a terminal prognosis. It's purpose is not to sugar-coat, not to trivialize, and not to frighten or frustrate you, but to provide straight talk to lessen your fear and improve your physical, emotional, and spiritual comfort. It was written to help you understand what can happen and what you can do about it. Not everyone wants to know, but if you are reading this, you are among the many patients who requested a direct answer to the question, "How will I die?"

Remember that although you are the person facing death, everyone who loves you will be impacted. Share this book with them. Discuss important issues and feelings. Good communication is an important part of adjusting to the changes that you and those around you are experiencing.

Each chapter in this book could be a small book in itself. I have chosen to keep the chapters short, at the risk of being overly simple, to introduce the topics in small and easily-digestible servings. There is ample information available in journals, in books, and on the Internet if you desire a deeper explanation on any subject. I also encourage you to utilize a hospice physician and hospice staff to provide more details about your specific circumstances.

You may not experience all of the symptoms and issues that are reviewed, and you may have others. Covering the most common causes and symptoms of declining health, I will also discuss how you and your loved ones can respond and provide the knowledge to help you "pack" for this most amazing and sometimes mysterious journey to your final destination.

My hope is that by the end of this book, you are able to take a deep breath and confidently declare, "It's not as scary as I thought—I can get through this!"

Your life may have been shorter than you wanted or anticipated, but for however many days or months remain, you still have life to be lived fully. There are still special moments to be experienced, and there is still love to be shared.

Your life is measured
not by the number of breaths you take,
but by the number of moments
that take your breath away.
—Author Unknown

YOUR WORLD HAS CHANGED

You've Been Given the Bad News—Now What?

Take a deep breath and breathe out slowly. Your doctor has just told you that you are in the final days or months of your life. What should you expect and how soon? Will death just show up, unannounced and without warning? Can you safely return to your car without suddenly collapsing? Will family members look at you nervously from across the table, wondering how many pillows they should place around your chair in case you fall over right there? Should you climb into bed now that this death sentence has been passed and just wait for it to be carried out? What are the road markers? What are the road hazards? Are there detours you can take? And what about that final destination …?

You're in new and frightening territory. Learning to live well has brought enough challenges. Now you have been told to change tracks and begin to die well. Where do you learn these skills that you'd really rather not have to obtain? Have you witnessed anyone else on this journey, and what has that taught you? Will you and your loved ones be willing and able students as you go through this? You can't run from it, but who wants to embrace dying? Isn't there a way to avoid this altogether?

> *Everybody has got to die, but I have always believed*
> *an exception would be made in my case.*
> —Author William Saroyan, on his deathbed

Intellectually you've always known that one day you will die, but somehow, it comes as a surprise. You just didn't expect it ... yet. There is rarely a good time to die. Since living forever is not an option, let's talk about the choices you *do* have.

Getting the Help You Need

You need not be alone in this process. Naturally, you will be filled with a lot of questions and fears. There are many myths and misconceptions about dying that may feed your fears. You need straight talk delivered honestly and compassionately. You need to be able to ask the most difficult questions without someone avoiding, minimizing, or trivializing them.

You may never have witnessed the death of someone close to you, so perhaps you can't begin to know what to expect. Or worse, you may have heard horror stories about someone's dying, which causes you to naturally believe that all death is horrible or involves pain. Your own doctor may not be able to specifically tell you what happens, because he/she has been trained to preserve life, not prepare people for death. So where do you go?

I recommend seeking the support of hospice right away. Available and able to respond twenty-four hours a day, seven days a week, a comprehensive hospice team understands that dying is not just a physical event, but that it will touch every aspect of life for both you and your family. The team is prepared to help you manage the physical, emotional, and spiritual challenges you and your family may face in your final months.

The hospice team includes your physician, a nurse, a social worker, a chaplain, a home-health aide, and a bereavement counselor. They make intermittent visits to your place of residence and are only a phone call away at all times. They are gentle guides, whose intention is to help you remain as comfortable and functional as you can within the limits of your particular disease. This comfort includes the provision of all necessary medication, equipment, and supplies related to your illness. Trained volunteers, physical, occupational and speech-language therapists, a nutritionist, and a pharmacist are also available as needed. Helping you maximize your life while you prepare for death, they will honor your beliefs and traditions, and support your family during this time and for thirteen months after your death. This comprehensive care and support is provided in your home, where 90 to 95 percent of hospice patients are able to remain until death, although many hospice programs have a facility which is available for short-term stays. This facility can be used for symptom control, a break for the family, or for the actual dying event.

Worried about cost? The most comprehensive Medicare program available, hospice is covered 100 percent. For those not under Medicare, most insurance companies will cover hospice services. No insurance? Most hospices will also provide care at no charge to you. There is no reason you shouldn't get the care and support that you and your family need and deserve to ensure the best possible quality of life.

You can't do anything about the length of your life,
but you can do something about its width and depth.
—Author Unknown

Putting Aside the Old Ways

Throughout our lives, whenever we have been seriously ill or had surgery, the conventional and appropriate wisdom has been to slowly build back up—to eat a little more, to exercise a little more each day, and to gain strength and rebuild our health. When dealing with a terminal illness, this way of thinking must be replaced with a new way if your comfort is the priority. In this new scenario, you as the patient are the expert we consult regarding what you can and cannot do. Only you know what it's like to be inside your body. Only you know the limits you find each day, which may also vary each day. Yes, I'm saying that you have the ultimate say! If I as caregiver want to ensure your comfort and decrease stress for both of us, I must accept what you tell me about your desire or ability to eat or be active. For your family, this may not be an easy change to make, because the idea of *not* pushing food and drink or not forcing you to exercise each day may seem neglectful.

Learning to Listen to Your Body

There is more wisdom in your body
than in your deepest philosophy.
—Friedrick Nietzcshe

Dying is a natural process. Your body has amazing wisdom built in to take care of you during this time. Just like it must go through certain stages to be born, it must also go through certain stages while it shuts down toward death. Your job is to learn what the natural and normal changes are that we don't want to interfere with, lest we inadvertently create more discomfort. When dying, it is time to begin to listen to your body—*really* listen and then respond accordingly. This is no time to ignore its pleas just because you may have spent your life doing that. It's time for true self-care.

You will also want to learn how to manage possible symptoms, such as pain, shortness of breath, constipation, anxiety, and the like. When you understand what is happening and, most importantly, how best to manage the changes, you will be less fearful and more relaxed with the process, and even feel a sense of empowerment and peace. One related issue is whether or not to use artificial fluid and nutrition, which we will cover shortly.

How Will I Die?

> *"I'm not afraid of dying—I just don't want*
> *to be there when it happens."*

This Woody Allen quotation reflects what many of my patients feel about the dying process. They have a belief about what does or does not happen after death, but have many concerns about what they will have to go through to get there.

Few health-care practitioners have been taught about the dying process in their training. Your best resources are well-trained hospice professionals, who will help you understand what dying may look and feel like for you. They know that dying from brain cancer is different than dying from other cancers, heart disease, kidney failure, Alzheimer's, or old age. In my experience, once I have honestly and completely responded to the question, "How will I die?" by gently describing the most commonly expected changes that you may experience related to your specific disease and how to understand and manage each one, the sense of relief is powerful. Your energy can now be less tied up in the pregnant fear of unanswered questions and misconceptions, and is more available to apply to living the life you have.

So let's talk about the "why's" and "what's" of the most common changes that you may encounter so you will feel better prepared.

Losses and Gains

Each symptom of a decline in health is a loss to be grieved. Each loss may also bring fear and resistance, because you or your loved ones may not like the idea that you are getting closer to the end of your life and that there's nothing any of you can do about it. It's natural to try and fight against the changes, to question them, and to push our old beliefs about regaining health and lengthening life. It's not a path that is gracefully accepted when sadness about the end of life, anger about the losses, and a sense of helplessness about the future are frequent companions along the way. Sometimes you can adjust fairly graciously, but you may also adjust through gritted teeth. This is not the time to expect super-humanness from yourself or others. We are simply human, with all our inherent frailties and flaws.

Be gentle with each other. Return to the key chapters that you need in this book to ensure that you are doing what is necessary to achieve comfort and quality of life.

Although you are experiencing losses, there are also gains to be had. People facing the end of their lives often find a keener awareness and appreciation of people and things that they didn't acknowledge or took for granted when they were healthy. Many tell me their priorities shift. It's no longer important that your daughter folds your laundry just your way, the "right way", but rather that she is simply present in your life, offering help. The muddy paw prints on your tiles are nothing compared to the loving companionship and unconditional love of your puppy. That annoying habit of your spouse cracking knuckles is now, strangely enough, an endearing sound that you will miss. Your physical world may grow small with ever-decreasing abilities, but for many, the emotional and spiritual world grows ever larger. Quality of life may be redefined as you find great satisfaction in receiving the care and attention of more family and friends than you ever imagined cared that much. It can be downright humbling!

Physical Changes
Changes in Activity—The Conflict Begins

"But you love to work in your shop ... why aren't you doing that anymore? Are you giving up? You can't just give up!"

"Don't just lie there and die—get out of bed! Take a walk ... sit in the living room ... something ... anything!"

The essence of these statements reveals the emotional attachments to maintaining health and normalcy and to resisting the obvious symptoms of a decline. One of the first symptoms is the change in activity levels. In the past, you have been able to recover from health crises by forcing yourself to do more each day and building up strength, but this is not the case when dealing with a terminal illness. It's not out of defiance that you tell your loved ones you don't want to get up. It's not because they don't care about how you feel that they are pushing you to do more than you feel you can. Each change and each loss brings it's own disruption. It may take awhile for everyone to regain his or her balance when it feels like the rug is being pulled out from under you. Be patient with each other and know that all of the disruption is based in the fact that no one wants change, especially one that is leading toward the end of life.

Establishing Priorities

Here's an analogy that I've found helpful in understanding and accepting your decreasing physical abilities. The energy you have each day is like a pile of coins in your hands. This is your energy allowance for the day. That's all you have to spend. When it's gone, it's gone. The questions to ask yourself are, "How do I want to spend my energy today?" and "What is most important or meaningful for me to do today?" If you push yourself to get up, shower, and walk to the table for breakfast, you may have spent all your energy in one fell swoop. Now you are even too tired to eat, so pushing yourself to be active, to do what you always *used* to be able to do, has actually worked against you.

In setting energy priorities, consider if you really need a shower each day, or if it's ok to use the wheelchair to go outside on the patio instead of walking there if that means preserving your energy for what you really want—an afternoon visiting your friends or family, or a trip to your favorite restaurant for your anniversary.

Everything takes energy, even sitting and visiting with friends. Family may feel rejected because visits may be restricted in length and because you just don't communicate like you used to. They may wonder if you now find sleeping preferable to visiting with them. To help them feel less put off, ask if they remember being in the hospital or feeling severely ill at home. Did they remember what it was like when well-meaning friends came by to "cheer them up?" What did they really want to tell them? "Please go away!"

It's not that you don't appreciate their love and good intentions. It's just that your energy is now turning inward, toward yourself, for your own preparation and well-being. Let them know this doesn't mean you don't love and appreciate them. You are simply tired. Just lying there, you may be exhausted. Suggest to them that you can still gratefully receive their love by having them leave messages or cards that you can read and re-read when you have the energy.

When you get to the point where getting out of bed seems to be a monumental chore or even a burden, a technique that I've found to help family members understand how hard this is for you is to ask them to check your pulse. Chances are it's faster than the normal sixty, perhaps reaching one hundred to one hundred and ten beats per minute or more. That's the pulse of someone running a marathon. So in your case, it's like you've been running for twenty-six miles and haven't stopped—that's how tired you are. Once your family members comprehend this, it's easier for them to understand that forcing you to get out of bed is not only above and beyond what is physically comfortable, but that in fact it will take energy from you, exhausting you even further, rather than building you up.

Energy Surges

There may be days when you have a sudden surge of energy, sometimes precipitated by a special event. For example, your long-time best friend is coming and you haven't seen him in five years. You are able to remain perked up, laugh, skip your nap, and even eat a bit more. The family may wonder now if you've just been faking it before or manipulating them into believing you were weaker than you really were in the days prior. But that's usually not true. Once the special event has passed, you may find yourself even more exhausted, with a real need to catch up on your rest. These energy surges are like a withdrawal of several days of your energy allowance. Once spent, payback forces you to seek longer and deeper periods of rest, sleeping more in the next few days.

You Just Gonna Sleep?

For many people, naps begin to increase in both frequency and length. It may be that your family sees you sleeping much of the day. This can be stressful for families who are increasingly and painfully aware that they are seeing your last weeks, days, or hours. They may even feel rejected and think, "You'd rather sleep than talk with me?" Hoping that it's not part of your physical decline, they may point to the use of medication as the cause, especially pain medication. They may want to cut the doses back, since you seem very comfortable. Please do not consider this without consulting your physician or your hospice team. The reason you are comfortable is that you have the right amount of the right pain medication. The reason you are sleeping is that your body is shutting down. This process happens to those patients who are taking no medications whatsoever. In addition to declining energy, changes in your metabolism also contribute to this increased sleeping. It may be low oxygen, high calcium, a liver or kidney shutdown, or many other causes that are part of the normal shutdown process.

Many patients have shared with me that during this time of increased sleep and changing levels of consciousness, "they visit the other side," "do a life review," or are in conversation with "those who have come to help" them. It's experienced as an important time of preparation.

When asked, most people I have met describe their preferred death as one in which they simply die in their sleep, so here's the good news. That's usually what happens. You sleep more and more until you slip into a coma, the length of which can be minutes to days. During this time, your body continues to shut down toward death. Essentially, you die in your sleep.

I Can Hear You!

Even when you don't have the energy to respond to your loved ones anymore, we've discovered that you are still aware of and can benefit from their presence and their loving conversation. Studies indicate that your hearing is the last sense to go. Thus, we encourage loved ones to talk to you, tell their favorite stories, and gain closure. This conversation offers two benefits: 1) A person can't tell a favorite story and not bring the feeling of that story to the present moment, so in the midst of the pain of knowing someone you love is soon to die, a smile appears to accompany the warm memories of a shared experience; 2) Hearing them tell these stories, you will know how you will be remembered. You may not be at the memorial service to hear what people are saying about you, but you get a preview now! How great is that?

Love is the only thing we carry with us when we go,
and it makes the end so easy.
—Louisa May Alcott

One More Bite

appetite is changing. You used to bring fear to the face of all-you-can-eat buffet owners, but now just a few bites of food seem to satisfy you. Food may not taste the same. Your craving for the more complex gourmet foods has left. In fact, you crave canned peaches, and you would never have considered eating them just five months ago! Your body is choosing simple foods. You may be losing weight. You hardly recognize the person in the mirror, and you see shock or concern on the faces of visitors who haven't seen you since last year.

A loss of appetite is a very emotionally-charged change and, as such, can be a difficult loss for your family to adjust to. Your loved ones may anxiously push high-protein shakes and nutritional supplements on you. When you push away your plate of food, they beg you to take another bite ... or two ... or ten. The fear is that you are going to starve to death, and therefore, death can be pushed away for a little longer if you can just eat a little more. They may feel they are being negligent by not force-feeding you or considering artificial means of providing nutrition. Let's make something very clear here. Lack of eating is not the cause of dying—it is a symptom of the dying.

Remember what I said earlier about changing our thinking when faced with a terminal illness? Eating more will not make you feel better, and may, in fact, make you feel worse. The bottom line is, "Are you comfortable with the amount you are eating?" If you are, then I, as caregiver, must accept that, lest I create more stress for both you and me. Now I'm assuming your physician has already treated potentially reversible causes of lack of appetite, such as nausea, pain, depression, mouth sores, and the like. If any of these problems are interfering with your meals, then let your physician know right away.

Why Eating Isn't What It Used to Be

There is a point in illness when the body's ability to use and process food begins to decrease. Your gastrointestinal tract slows down and is less efficient. To force down food when your body says, "Please don't," may cause cramping, bloating, or even throwing up.

In the case of cancer, a chemical has been released in your body that blocks your desire to eat—that's your body's way of keeping you comfortable. It has also blocked the body's ability to store fat and protein, so even if you were force-fed, your body would not benefit from it. Here's where the wisdom of the body must be followed. Your body knows that there is one type of cell that *will* continue to feed, and that's the cancer cell. If we feed the cancer cell, we feed its growth. A larger tumor can create more discomfort. You and your body don't want that.

Another line of defense and comfort that your body has created is that in not eating much, your body goes into a process called ketosis. This stimulates a release of your natural endorphins, our internal "morphine," to promote a sense of well-being. Follow what your body tells you, and it will help keep you more comfortable.

Are you thinking about artificial nutrition, such as tube-feeding? There is certainly a place for that. If you feel hunger and simply can't eat because of difficulty swallowing due to a stricture or obstruction, then go for it! But once hunger is no longer felt, that's a sign from your body. Did you know that for those with severe debility and weight loss due to a stroke or Alzheimer's, the use of tube-feeding not only does not prolong life, but in many cases actually hastens death due to the complications of this intervention? The risk of aspiration, pneumonia, or complications due to immobility actually increases.

You may think, "Well, since I can't eat, I should at least take my vitamins." Without decent food and fluid intake, those vitamins won't be absorbed, so they won't be of use to you. To the contrary, they may actually create more distress by causing nausea.

How do you cut down the pressure of well-meaning but scared loved ones who are pushing food? Know that they love you, that they want you to be around as long as possible, and that they are feeling pretty darned helpless right now. None of you can change what is happening. You are going to die, and they are unhappy about that. They want to know if there is something they can offer to improve your quality of life, and traditionally we show nurturing and love by offering food. This is especially common in women, with them making proclamations such as, "Eat, eat ... you'll feel better." Gently tell them that eating makes you uncomfortable, but that it would be really nice if they could provide you with a loving and nurturing activity that will enhance your life while helping them feel useful and less helpless. Examples of services they could provide are giving you a massage, combing your hair, showing you a photo album, or playing some music for you. You may all benefit from this change in focus.

Dying of Thirst?

It's bad enough that you and your family have had to face the decline in activity and eating, but now the lack of drinking is seen as a more serious threat, as people instinctively understand that death is getting closer. Fear shows its head again as your family frets that you will die of thirst.

Some people have heard that dehydration is painful, so let me clarify this. Indeed, the dehydration of an otherwise healthy individual who is lost in the desert and has run out of water is not comfortable. Cramping, nausea, and even seizures may occur. But at the end of life, as the result of disease or old age, a person goes through a process called natural dehydration. Most people will declare they are perfectly comfortable. They will simply seek sips of fluid or ice chips, or they may be comforted by good mouth care.

A dry mouth does not necessarily mean dehydration. This dryness is often the result of narcotics or other medications. Studies have also shown that a dry mouth is not relieved, even with artificial hydration.

You are the expert on what your body really needs to maintain comfort. It's amazing how little food and drink a person can survive on for weeks or months. As long as you are comfortable, that is all we can seek.

The Benefit of Natural Dehydration

Not wanting extra fluid right now is also your body's way of protecting itself. Remember when I told you that your heart may be working hard, which is reflected in a higher-than-normal pulse rate when you are resting? Well, it's the heart that has to handle fluid in your body. If someone starts an intravenous now to provide more fluid, the heart says, "Wait! How am I supposed to handle all this extra work? I'm working pretty hard as it is!" It may begin to store the fluid in parts of your body, which results in the swelling of your feet, hands, and backside. At worst, fluid may back up into your lungs and create more problems.

The ways in which natural dehydration benefits you are many. There are less gastric secretions, and therefore less chance of nausea and vomiting, less ascites (abnormal fluid collection in your belly), less swelling in your extremities (which puts you at risk of a bedsore), less lung congestion, and less frequency of incontinence (inability to hold your urine). Your body, in its infinite wisdom, has put dehydration in place to keep you comfortable, and it also stimulates those wonderful endorphins to promote a sense of well-being.

Of Bowels and Bladders

The goal here is to keep everything functioning as .. .... possible. If you are on narcotics, you should also be on a bowel program of softeners and mild stimulants to counteract their effect. Narcotics slow down the movement of your intestines. Combine that with less activity and less fluid intake, and you have a recipe for serious constipation. Even if you are barely eating or just drinking now, your body will continue to produce waste. A little bit of waste can create a hard little "rock" in your intestines. This can create bloating, cramping, nausea, and even make you want to stop your pain medications altogether. Know that constipation is a very manageable symptom that your hospice team takes very seriously. You do not want to go more than three days without a bowel movement. Trust me.

If you are at the place where natural dehydration has begun, your urine will become more concentrated, appearing darker in color and with a stronger smell. That's normal and nothing to worry about. If you no longer have the warning you need to urinate in a toilet, adult briefs/diapers can be used, or a catheter can be inserted. A catheter is a flexible tube that drains urine continuously from your bladder into a bag. One benefit is that it keeps you from having to get on and off the toilet or bedpan when you are feeling so weak. It will also keep you from getting wet and necessitating frequent bed and clothing changes.

Breathing Easier

Perhaps you are anemic, or you have heart or lung disease. You may experience dwindling energy. It may be that you can't concentrate as you once did and seem to get short of breath too easily with minimal activity. It may be that you feel a bit restless without knowing why—especially at night, which causes you to loose precious sleep. A lowered oxygen level in your body can be the cause of all of these symptoms.

While the use of oxygen is common and very useful under these circumstances, the acceptance that you must now wear tubing on your face and cart around a machine is a bit tough for some, at least initially. With the oxygen equipment as a constant tethered companion, there is a visible sign of decline and of frailty, and you may sense a loss of freedom. It's another adjustment.

Let's look at how it can benefit you. First, adequate oxygen will cut down the stress on your body. You will sleep better, have an increased attention span, require fewer naps, move around more, and remain independent longer. These are all good things, so don't be afraid to try it. It's OK to start slowly, if that's important to you, and to take the time to adjust to it. Keep it on before, during, and after your bath time and other activities, or for a half-day. Try to notice the difference it makes, and ask your caregivers what they notice. For some, it's a huge and wonderful difference, while for others, it's more subtle but still significant in fine-tuning your quality of life.

You need the oxygen the most when you are active, so please don't remove it to take your shower or go shopping. Your heart and lungs won't have to work so hard if you have oxygen along with the right medications to help you breathe well.

If it adds to your safety and quality of life, why not make your oxygen equipment one of your best companions?

Fear of Suffocating

If you have been experiencing a disease in which your breathing has been affected, it's understandable to believe that it will only get worse until the moment of death, and that at that moment, you will be gasping for air. The good news is that your body's wisdom and protective mechanisms will kick in to assure your comfort.

If you have difficulty breathing months and days before the end, your physician can order medications and treatments that will help you relax and breathe easier. This is important to relieving your fear. Anxiety can worsen the feeling of being short of breath, so we often treat both. The use of medication, oxygen, calming music, relaxation techniques, or a small fan blowing on the side of your face are all tools that can benefit you.

When you get very close to death, the amount of oxygen in your body will naturally decrease. If you are in a hospital, the staff may be measuring this change and responding by increasing your oxygen rate, even though your comfort level hasn't changed. I highly recommend that they do not adjust your oxygen in the absence of any distress, because they may actually be unknowingly prolonging dying and creating discomfort. Your body has a mechanism that, when allowed, will keep you comfortable. When the oxygen in your body gets low enough and the carbon dioxide in your system builds up, it's called oxygen narcosis, which promotes a sense of calm as you slip into a coma. When this happens, all struggles leave you, and you breathe easier. You will essentially have "gone to sleep," and your loved ones will be happy to see easier breathing and no agitation. Increasing the oxygen or using a high-tech oxygen mask will only delay this natural and peaceful process.

Your breathing patterns might change now, though you will be unaware of this. Your family may see irregular, shallow, or deep breathing. Anything that is not the norm might make them worry that you are struggling. Your relaxed face will help assure them that you are fine.

What's That Noise?

When your swallow and cough reflex stops as you get close to death, fluid begins to collect on top of your larynx. As you breathe, this fluid bubbles with the air exchange and can create a noise that some call the death rattle. Even though you as the patient are comfortable and not struggling, this noise can be very distressing to the family. A change in position can be tried. Suctioning is not recommended, because it's invasive and the fluid will just recollect. If the noise is coming from deeper in your lungs because fluid has built up there, there are medications to dry up those secretions. At this point, you may be minimally conscious, but you're more likely comfortably in a coma and completely unaware.

Thankfully, the death rattle is not common. Because it is distressing to hear, I suggest distracting noise. My preferred recommendation is to get the family to start talking to you or about you and to share stories, laughter, and tears. That deep sharing benefits all involved, because it facilitates grieving and closure.

Don,t have more to say? I'll recommend music. This is a time to play music or sounds that they know *you* love. I have told my sons that if they play rap music at my deathbed, I will come back to haunt them! And please *leave* the TV *off*. During the time of dying, and you don't need to be reminded about the war, the economy and the like. But if you find comfort in hearing your favorite basketball team playing, as my mother-in-law did the day before she died, then so be it. Be sure your family knows what music you like—or a preferred reading—or silence.

Dying of heart failure, James responded neither to voice nor touch for the past 3 days as he drifted deeper into his coma. His wife, Edith, sought the comfort of her favorite music, and soon lyrics of Boccelli's Favorite Hits filled the room. James suddenly opened his eyes and exclaimed, "I hate Boccelli!" and faded back into his coma.

Confusion Can Be Confusing

Confusion can be caused by the process of the body shutting down and by the dying itself. This is when your family will benefit from the assessment of a good health-care provider. Often the family will suspect medications as the probable culprit. Can some medications cause confusion? Yes. If that is the case, your physician can work with you to adjust or change those meds. But more often, confusion is due to natural body changes that are disease specific, like decreasing oxygen, failing liver and kidneys, a high calcium level from bone metastasis, brain swelling, or other metabolic changes.

In addition to the natural physical changes, there may be other changes in awareness and consciousness that look confusing. As some people have described it to me, there's a sense that you are visiting one world when you are sleeping, and when you awaken back into this one, it can be disorienting. Sometimes you may see things that no one else does, but I'll discuss visions and final messages a bit later. Ask your hospice nurse about the possible causes of confusion and what, if anything, can realistically be done.

About Those Eyes

As you sleep or drift into a coma, it may be that your eyelids no longer completely close. Family may wonder if you are trying to remain conscious. What's happening is that the fat pad that is behind the eye begins to shrink due to dehydration. The eyes are simply falling back further into your head. The image may create some distress for observers, but when the dynamics are understood, it's easier to accept when the lids will no longer close. Eyes drops can keep your eyes moist and comfortable.

Cold Feet and Other Symptoms

As your body continues to shut down, there are a number of changes that may occur. Remember how I said the heart was working hard to keep up with the changes? There's a time when it declares, "Enough work, already! I can only handle so much! So I'm gonna make sure blood gets to the most important parts—the brain, lungs, and kidneys. Arms and legs, you're just not that critical, so I'm cutting you off." As a result of this shift in circulation, your feet and hands become colder. Your family may see red or purple blotching on the soles of your feet and palms of your hands, which we call mottling. There is a tendency to want to cover you with blankets to "keep you warm," but even in a coma, you may instinctively kick them off. Not only do you not feel cold, but in fact, you may feel hot and even run a fever. The blood that is being concentrated in your torso gives you that feeling. Encourage your family to pay attention to what keeps you comfortable. If you kick off the blankets, they stay off. You remain the expert in what is needed.

Pain Is Not Inevitable

Did you know that many people die without any pain whatsoever, never taking so much as an aspirin? It is often mistakenly believed that pain naturally accompanies dying. This is simply not true. It is also not true that if pain is a part of your disease, you must learn to suffer in silence.

It is never, ever acceptable for your health-care provider to say, "I'm sorry, there is nothing more I can do about your pain ... you will have to learn to live with it."

Such a statement simply means that person does not have the training and skills needed to successfully manage your pain. Know that *all* pain can be managed. There are several types of pain and many types of medications. It takes the right drug or right combination of drugs for your particular pain. If your health-care team is lacking in this specialized knowledge, your best course of action is to find a physician in a pain clinic or one who is board certified in hospice and palliative care. Advances are being made all the time. You deserve to be comfortable.

Why Pain Is Your Enemy

Uncontrolled pain releases damaging stress hormones that further harm your body. Pain distances you from your world and the people you care about. Pain limits your ability to do the things you want and to participate as fully as possible in your life. Pain robs you of hope, of your personhood, and of your ability to move, to breathe, to actively engage in your life, and to share important times with your loved ones. The physical, psychological, social, and spiritual consequences of unrelieved pain can be enormous for both you and your family. You must insist on excellent pain control.

Dispelling the Myths about Pain Medications

You may have heard scary stories about morphine and the use of other narcotics. Too many people believe their only choices are suffering with pain, receiving narcotics and getting too drugged up to know what is happening, or hastening their death. These are common misconceptions or misinterpretations about what is truly occurring.

Will pain medications cause you to become incompetent or rob you of your final days of life? The answer is no! What will rob you of living well is inadequate pain management. A study published in the Journal of Hospice and Palliative Care in December of 2006 reports that patients actually live longer in hospice because their distressing symptoms are managed. Now, it's true that if someone suddenly increased your pain medications to ten times your previous dose, that may hasten your death. But good hospice workers, in conjunction with your physician, are trained in how to gradually increase doses, if and when needed, using well-established and published guidelines. Therapeutic dosages will not hasten dying. Therapeutic dosages will, in fact, add to your quality of life. I've had a number of patients who were homebound or even bed bound due to uncontrolled pain or breathing problems. Once on the right dose of a narcotic, they were able to get up and rejoin life, enjoying their hobbies again and even traveling!

But what about those stories you've heard, when someone started receiving morphine and then soon died? It's not uncommon that even doctors and nurses buy into this myth when they have not had adequate training in pain management. Some people incorrectly believe that a morphine drip is just an unofficially acceptable, under-the-table form of euthanasia. It would indeed be frightening to believe that health-care professionals are hastening your death under the guise of comfort. The real story is that, sadly, too many people receive adequate symptom management only when they are within days or hours of dying. The morphine that could have benefited them for months is now only provided on their deathbed. The person was already in the process of dying. The morphine just kept them comfortable while that natural process continued.

There is the rare occurrence of what is called intractable pain. That is pain that we are unable to relieve and still assure consciousness. In my thirty years as a RN, I've only seen this three times. If a patient is close to death and all other pain therapies have been tried without success, then the option of sedation is considered. The person is medicated only to the point of sedation sufficient to relieve pain without hastening death. Narcotics are not used to produce these sedative effects, though they will continue to be used for pain management.

Because this choice is only available when you are close to death and you have chosen to be rendered unconscious to avoid the experience of pain, this intervention is easily misunderstood as euthanasia or hastening death. Studies have found that there is no difference in survival of those who required sedation in the final days versus those who did not. We can periodically allow the medications to wear off to offer the patient food and drink and again ask if he/she prefers consciousness or wants to resume sedation.

Narcotics not only relieve pain but also help you breathe better. They don't stop your breathing, as another myth proclaims, and they can actually improve it! When close to death, if people are fighting pain or shortness of breath, they are also fighting dying. With the proper medications, that struggle may be replaced with comfort, peace, and letting go. Did the narcotic hasten their death? No, it made their journey toward death more comfortable. In hospice, we honor the natural process of dying, neither postponing nor hastening death.

When Addiction Is the Fear

"I'll get addicted if I use narcotics."
"Who cares if he gets addicted—he's dying!"

While the above statements are often heard from patients, families, and even health-care professionals, they are also based on misinformation and fear. The possibility of addiction in people who have no prior history of abuse is exceedingly rare. Because of the phenomenally low rate of addiction in the terminally ill who have pain, it should not be an issue. The greater concern is that this fear may keep you from reaching good pain control.

Addiction refers to the use of medications for nonmedical purposes, usually with harm to the individual. It applies when a person has no pain but uses narcotics to get a high. That's a nontherapeutic use, meaning you are using the narcotics for something other than their intended purpose. But if you are having pain, you need pain medication—period. Whether you need these medications for three days or thirty years, it cannot be considered an addiction when you are treating your pain so you can enjoy an improved quality of life.

What If I Have a History of Addiction?

If you have overcome previous addictions to alcohol or drugs, you may be fearful your addiction will be triggered again. You may have a tendency to avoid pain medications altogether by toughing it out. Your family may express their fear about you using the pain medications and may even try to keep you from using them.

If you have pain, you deserve to have that pain relieved, whether you have been or are currently a drug user for nonmedicinal reasons. It may be that with your history of drug use, your tolerance for medications is now high, and you will therefore need a higher dose of drug than the average person. In hospice, we worry less about the dosage, and more about whether it's effective or not. If you are currently using drugs recreationally for nonmedicinal purposes, then your health-care team will work closely with you to set therapeutic guidelines.

The necessary dosages can vary greatly with the individual, the disease, and the length of time he/she has been on pain medications. I've had patients receiving one milligram of morphine every four hours and those receiving one thousand milligrams every hour. These are huge difference in doses, but in each case, the patient was alert and walking around. The particular dosage for each individual was what was required to achieve comfort and promote optimal function. Your physician and hospice team will work closely with you and your family to determine what you need.

SECTION TWO

Choices and Control

To Treat or Not to Treat

The decision to allow a natural death, to refuse artificial nutrition and hydration, to refuse to be treated for pneumonia or a urinary tract infection other than to manage symptoms, or to refuse dialysis or ventilators *is not an act of negligence.* It is an act of love. Just because we have technology doesn't mean we are required to use it if it only creates or prolongs suffering. The question to keep asking is if we are prolonging living or prolonging dying. Determining the desired goals and the impact of those goals must be discussed with your physician or hospice team.

> *It is the duty of a physician to prolong life.*
> *It is not his duty to prolong dying.*
> —Lord Thomas Horder, 1936

You have the right to choose—always. Sometimes choices are clear. Sometimes the emotions generated by you and your loved ones create a muddiness you can't see through. Perhaps you have lung cancer, ALS (Lou Gerhig's Disease), or Alzheimer's disease, and you get a bout of pneumonia. Pneumonia was once considered "the old man's friend," because it was a common and natural death. The terminal phase was comparatively short, and people knew what to expect and how to maintain comfort. But nowadays it's also very treatable. Be assured that without antibiotic treatment, the symptoms are very manageable to maintain your comfort, so the question arises, "Is it in your best interest to treat the pneumonia?" Perhaps you were fairly strong prior to the infection, and this is a bump in the road that you can get by fairly well. A course of antibiotics may be desirable and reasonable in this case. But perhaps you were experiencing a high level of deterioration or incapacitation prior to the pneumonia, and treating it may only assure that you will continue to experience this decreased level of health. The pneumonia may come back at a later point, too. You may prefer to let nature takes its course and focus on comfort only.

> *Death, taxes, and childbirth. There's never any*
> *convenient time for any of them.*
> —Margaret Mitchell

As health-care workers, it's not our job to tell you what to do. Our job is to educate you on the benefits and burdens of any decision, to provide information about how we will manage your symptoms, with or without more aggressive treatment, and to provide the emotional support you and your family will need as you navigate this time of decision-making. There will usually be doubts, second-guessing, and fears as you wonder if you are all doing the right thing to treat or not treat. The truth is, no matter what your age or your level of debility, family is hardly ever ready to lose you, often seeking another week or another month. You, yourself, despite feeling so incapacitated, may also not be ready to let go of life. This is when you can truly benefit from outside support to make sure that whatever decision you make, it truly reflects your goals, beliefs, and values and is not based on guilt, fear, lack of information, or misinformation.

Promises and Pitfalls of Experimental Therapies

I don't want to achieve immortality through my work;
I want to achieve immortality through not dying.
—Woody Allen

The promise of a possibly longer life with experimental therapy has to be weighed against the possibility of an impaired quality of life or even a shortened life due to complications. Especially in the case of cancer, by the time you are offered the chance to participate in a trial drug study, your disease is usually fairly advanced, and although there is no longer the hope of a cure, there may be hope of extended life. You may also want to find value in and to contribute to a field of science to help patients in the future, based on your reactions now. This is the time to look closely at what you may still want to experience in your life and how this treatment might impact that.

Roger and Christine loved to travel and did so frequently in their thirty-five years of marriage. This pattern was disrupted several times in the past few years as Roger dealt with the diagnosis of esophageal cancer and the resultant treatments. No longer responding to chemotherapy, he was offered an experimental therapy, which had only a slight chance of offering an extended life, but a greater chance of side effects that could actually detrimentally affect his quality of life. He and his wife talked at length about their wishes for their final weeks or months together. They had missed traveling in the past eight months due to his treatments. They worked together to balance their needs and goals in life with treatment options. Roger wanted any chance at extending his life. After some discussion with his hospice nurse and physician, he decided to opt for the experimental treatment, but only after enjoying a final cruise with his wife to Alaska, their favorite destination. Blood transfusions and pain management were provided to promote his comfort so they could enjoy their trip, creating wonderful lasting memories for Christine. Upon his return, he planned to sign out of the hospice program to receive the experimental therapy.

When they returned from their trip, Roger decided against the experimental therapy after all. They had enjoyed their trip and talked and cried as they reviewed their lives together. He felt content about his life and opted not to leave Christine with final memories of difficult side effects. He knew he could always change his mind, but felt his battle was over. He wanted to enjoy his final time in comfort, even if it meant fewer days or weeks.

The choice is yours.

Stan was proud of his years as a lab researcher. His enthusiasm and commitment to his work left him no time to develop relationships outside of his work, and so he never married and had no friends outside of his workplace. An only child, his parents had immigrated from Poland, where most of his family had been killed in the Holocaust. So when he was diagnosed with pancreatic cancer, Stan was focused on the latest trials of experimental drugs. Despite the fact that there was little chance of a remission of his cancer, he found tremendous interest and value in "being a guinea pig," as he described it, and let his doctors know of his hope that his case would be written up in a journal. That was the legacy he chose.

This decision-making is rarely easy. Your heart and mind may be at odds, not to mention those of your family and friends. Honoring life, promoting comfort, and listening to your body as your best guide are all important. Yet advances in technology have changed the culture of dying and have fed the belief that we can push away death. Technology is seductive, with its teasing promise that each little decline or complication can be reversed, causing us to lose sight of the fact that regardless of the small battles, there's still a big war that will eventually be lost. Is your definition of the "good fight" battling every skirmish until the end, using whatever treatments you can find to get another day, week, or month? Or is the "good fight" simply acceptance of the inevitable with grace, putting your energies not into battle, but into living comfortably and finding closure? It's your choice. Consider the benefits and burdens to yourself and your family, physically, emotionally, spiritually, and even financially. How might your decision impact how you want to spend your final weeks or months? With what memories will you leave your family? What will they learn from your dying? How will that help them as they prepare for their own death in the future?

A good death does honor to a whole life.
—Petrarch

About Those Questions of Control

"I just want to stay in control—that's all! "

This is not an uncommon desire of those who are as fearful as living as they are of dying. Can you control your dying? Dying itself is a process of letting go, so if you are inclined to be a control freak, this may not be easy. You will be challenged. You may be awed. You may experience a full range of emotions: anger, denial, guilt, joy, acceptance, frustration, and peace—sometimes within the course of minutes! Can you transcend the losses and challenges to your being and find new meaning and value in your life? Yes. Can fear and frustration be transformed into a state of grace and acceptance? Yes. Can you swing back into fear and frustration an hour later? Yes. Everything is possible in this very dynamic process.

Accept your own humanness and that of your family. You're not going to get through this looking good. There is no one course, "right way," or perfect death. Everyone will idealize their image of a "good death" and should have the opportunity to bring their individual definition to the table to be shared, so in the end, there is a sense of acceptance and satisfaction that you all understood and did the best you could under difficult circumstances. Continually forgiving yourself and forgiving others is often critical work on this journey.

Life is an adventure in forgiveness.
—Norman Cousins

The Big Challenge

Often lying just behind our desire for control and independence is the belief or fear that we only have value because of what we *do*—as a teacher, lawyer, mother, inventor, writer, everyone's favorite cook, or the person who is always helping others. Doing tasks is what we often believe gives us value and meaning, which we too often seek in the eyes of others, not ourselves. So what happens when you are no longer *doing*? Are you worthy of someone's love and care just for *being*? You may be used to being the giver, but now you are forced into the uncomfortable role of receiver, and you wonder if you are worthy of this, since you are no longer contributing in the ways you used to. You search the eyes of those caring for you, wondering how they see you now. Do they feel burdened? Do they really want to do this? You may challenge them and test them to see their reaction. You don't like ending on a low note, not continuing to be the source of strength and power that you are used to being. You worry that their last image of you may be of a fading star, not a shining one.

If this matches your perception or fear, can we agree to put it aside for a moment while we look at what is also possible now?

Receiving as a Gift

"'Tis better to give then receive" is a common belief that needs to be gently set aside right now, even though that may be difficult. Many of us are very comfortable with the role of always giving and always helping. We hope people will be grateful receivers of what we offer. But will we ask for help for ourselves? No way! The very idea makes us grimace and step back. That would change our image of ourselves! We've never asked for help, and we certainly don't want to start now! What would people think of us? Wouldn't we be considered weak, pathetic, or something much worse?

So let's rethink this. When you offered your help, strength, or experience to another, did you consider them weak or incapable? Or did you simply want to be of service? How did you feel if they rejected your well-intentioned offer of help? How did it feel if they gratefully accepted? Didn't it feel good to be able to offer something to someone you cared about? Wasn't it particularly sweet if you discovered that you could make a difference? Well, why would you want to deny that feeling now to those who love you and want to show you that love? In learning the fine art of receiving graciously, you are actually giving! You are giving them the chance to return favors and to show you they care. The circle of giving and receiving is finally complete. It is in giving that we receive and in receiving that we give. Allow it. It's not a time for ego, but for gratitude and appreciation.

Are you worried about being a burden or that your loved ones have better things to do? I have to let you know about the real sense of gratitude that families have expressed for the chance to provide care. Was it easy? No. Did it provide valuable life lessons? Yes. Did they regret being a caregiver? No! In their grief they were comforted by knowing they did the best job possible. They expressed a sense of pride and accomplishment, grateful to have those final memories and the chance to show how much they loved the person they cared for.

Learn to receive and allow those who love you to have the opportunity to give. Who you are is not diminished by this process, but enhanced.

Letting Go

Who doesn't like the illusion of being in control? Haven't we run much of our lives with the belief that if things just happened the way we wanted or planned, then everything would have been better? But life keeps happening while we make plans, and as human beings we have an amazing capacity to adjust and move on—gracefully at times, kicking and screaming at other times. No one said we'd get through life looking good. But our lessons, our wounds, and our victories have all sculpted us into the magnificent form we currently are. We survived the changes. We grew from our experiences. Dying is our last chapter. Dying itself is a process of letting go and a key lesson in this final chapter.

Some people have an especially hard time letting go of life and the illusion of control that they've sought for so many years, through marriage, children, career, and the like. There's some sneaky and yet undiscovered gene that makes us feel responsible for everyone else within our realm, and this belief is not shaken, even when we are facing our death. It seems we are never released from this self-inflicted responsibility.

Who wants to believe the world can move on without them? Would that mean we didn't make a real difference? "But I've worked so hard," you might say. Sometimes we inadvertently create a dependency by always taking over, so our children, spouses, or co-workers learn they can't possibly make decisions on their own—certainly not the right ones! "See," you proclaim, "I can't leave now! They need more help! I have to make sure everything is tied up perfectly before I can leave this earth." Somehow we feel responsible for the feelings and choices of others. The good news, or the bad news, depending on how you look at it, is that you are not responsible. You can't control what they are experiencing. We can love, nurture, direct, hope, and pray. What wonderful gifts to offer! The other person will decide what to do or not do with those gifts, and there's not a darn thing you can do about it. So letting go is really just finally acknowledging the reality that you didn't really have control in the first place!

Will there be pain and sadness upon your death? Yes. Can you do anything to prevent that pain and sadness? No. Pain is the cost of loving someone who someday must leave you. You can't prevent their sadness any more than you can prevent your own, knowing you will no longer be a part of their day-to-day living on the physical plane. Your lives have been woven together, and your shared times will always be a part of that person's heart.

What you leave behind is not
what is engraved in stone monuments,
but what is woven into the lives of others.
—Pericles

But I Still Want Control

So isn't there *something* you can control? Certainly. You can control your own reactions, but not anyone else's. Just how you choose to experience the changes toward your impending death—how you prepare, how you participate, and how you love—is completely within your control.

No Need to Lose Your Dignity

The ideal man bears the accidents of life with dignity and grace,
making the best of circumstances.
—Aristotle

The fear inspired by the inability to be self-sufficient, the possibility you may eventually require help with basic needs, and the thought that you may lose control of your body's waste, tends to activate nervous twitches in many people. Too often it is considered one of the most dreaded insults to our dignity. Your ego may certainly take a hit, but your dignity is who you are, how you respond to changes, and how you rise above to face challenges. No one can take that from you. It has nothing to do with whether you are able to wipe your own face or behind. Dignity cannot be taken by someone else unless you surrender it yourself. Dignity is defined as, "The quality of being worthy of esteem or respect." Surrender, humility, and love are all aspects of dignity, which is yours to keep.

"Sure," you may be thinking, "it's easy for you to say this because, as a nurse, you're on the preferred side of the bed rails." But take it from someone who knows. I encourage you to read Mitch Ablom's *Tuesdays With Morrie,* a true story about a man with ALS (Lou Gerhig's Disease). As he was eventually unable to do anything for himself because of the progressive debilitation of this neurological disease, he transcended his attachments to *doing* and reveled in just *being.* In this state of being, he graciously and even enthusiastically received the loving care and attention of others. Now, you may be reading this and saying, "Good for him, but that's not for me!" I understand. I don't relish the idea of losing my independence, either. I doubt anyone does. I ask you to just consider the idea that illness is transformative and that we make ongoing adjustments. As our physical world becomes limited, our emotional and spiritual worlds can become limitless.

An act of surrender is needed—surrendering to the process of dying and all that it entails. It can also invoke a sense of humility to let go of that over which we have no control and accept the changes. I have witnessed the amazing grace of countless patients who let go of their previous self-image and focused on what was most important—giving and receiving love.

The Line in the Sand

We admire the death of leaves,
why not our own?
—Tom Bahti

"If I can't walk on my own power, life isn't worth living!"

Again and again, I've watched as the "line in the sand" that people proclaim they never want to cross and never plan to cross begins to shift. Herein lies the transformation that is possible in illness. You may declare that life isn't worth living if you can't travel the world anymore, but you soon begin to discover the beauty of your neighborhood and your own home and find contentment there. Early on, the idea of a wheelchair makes you cringe, yet you eventually begin to see it as your best friend, because with it, you still have the ability to visit your friends, go to the store or church, and sit on the patio. You are initially adamant about your privacy and independence, but eventually discover you look forward to the bed baths and massage that your spouse or the nurse's assistant provides. You even discover that adult diapers are really rather convenient! Things you never thought would be acceptable when you were healthier are now just a series of minor adjustments, because you continue to redefine your values and discover new meaning in life. You may have fewer choices, but you still have choices about the little things that make up your day and how you perceive your life. It's less about focusing on what you have lost and more about accepting and appreciating what you still have.

Alex was in the end stages of AIDS. Having seen his partner and several friends die of the disease, he knew what he may be facing. Alex drew a line in the sand, announcing his demands to his hospice nurse.

Several months passed, and that line in the sand was eventually crossed without incident, becoming just a memory. Wanting to explore his current perceptions and plans, his nurse reminded him of their previous conversation. "Oh that!" Alex said with a sheepish grin, "I finally decided that killing myself would be like skipping the last class."

This earth is a giant classroom, and we are perpetual students. As we go through life, we face many difficulties. Those who advance the idea of assisted suicide may declare that dying is one difficult challenge that should be avoided because the end of life may be stressful and messy, and everyone loses sleep. Have you had children? Wasn't it messy and stressful, and didn't you lose sleep when they were babies? How about when they were teenagers? Well, my three sons were teenagers at the same time, and although it was a challenge, I let all of us live! When we make it through the challenging times, we hopefully grow in wisdom, in understanding, and in tolerance. We gain strength. We are shaped by our experiences. So why would we "skip the last class" when often our most important life lessons arrive near the end, for patient and family alike? When we receive the support and love we need to make it through the difficult times, it makes a world of difference.

If Thoughts Turn to Suicide

Fears are powerful, and they tend to be worse than reality. Dread, fear, misinformation, and lack of information can contribute to a person desiring a hastened death. Unrelieved and uncomfortable symptoms and depression can also cause this line of thinking. If you are wishing for a hastened death, I ask you to do two things: 1) Make sure all your symptoms are under control. Life looks differently when you are comfortable; 2) Find out if you are suffering from depression. Sadness is different from depression, and you will need a clinician to diagnose and treat this. Don't try to beat a hasty exit from this world when there's something positive that can still be done for you.

Suicidal thoughts are not uncommon when facing a terminal condition, so don't be afraid to talk to your hospice team about them. If you are having these thoughts, my questions are "What do you fear the most?" and "What in particular would make you feel you want a hastened death?" Very often it's the lack of information or misinformation that precipitates these thoughts, and voicing your concerns gives the hospice team a chance to respond to them. Is it fear of pain? Make sure your hospice team will provide good pain control and that you learn to communicate your needs.

"I just don't want to be a burden on my family."

This is the second-most common concern in my experience. Please review the chapters on communication, receiving, and the line in the sand. Discuss your concern with your family and remain open to their responses. Discuss it with your hospice team and let them work with you and your family. While suicide may seem like an easier and more painless way to exit your life, please consider the impact on your family. Consider the process of dying, letting go, and allowing the transformation of illness to take place. Again and again, I've had patients who strongly desired suicide when their disease got to a certain point, and each time, the line in the sand moved. Let me talk about how and why that can happen by sharing a lesson a patient revealed to me years ago.

Tom was sixty-two when he was diagnosed with prostate cancer. He was offered a definitive cure if he opted for surgery, but it ran the risk of rendering him impotent. Since Tom had just married his twenty-nine year old wife, Sandy, he declared, "No way! This is my life, I will run it the way I see fit, and disability will never be a part of that!" Tom was the kind of patient that scared most nurses. When he pushed his nurse's call light, he also pushed the button on his stopwatch and would let the nurse know how long it took her to respond. He was a man who was used to being in control, giving orders, and expecting others to respond. He didn't like surprises. He was proud of the business he built up by himself. He would talk with me about his disease and simply declare, "If this cancer gets to be a problem, I'm taking my life. Being ill is not an acceptable option to me." In my youth and inexperience, I just nodded, because in truth, I felt the same way. It was years later that I recognized that anyone needing that level of control was also very scared.

Over the next two years, Tom came back to the hospital again and again. Each time the cancer had progressed. Each time he opted for further intervention, and each time, he restated his declaration, "If this cancer gets to be a problem, I'm going to take those pills." He had stockpiled pills at home and even let his physician know his suicidal intentions.

A few months later, upon hearing that he was not doing well, I visited Tom and Sandy in their small apartment.

A hospital bed filled the small living room, and Tom lay propped up on one elbow. He was now paralyzed from the waist down because the tumor had damaged his spine. He had tubes inserted into his kidneys because his bladder had been removed, and urine was draining into a bag on the floor. He had lost control of his bowels, and because of the frequent diarrhea, he was developing sores on his buttocks. He was dry heaving into a bucket that he held under his chin, and he had painful spasms every twenty seconds or so. It was not a pretty picture and certainly not how I ever expected to see Tom. I sat down so we could be at eye level, and I said, "Well, Tom, it looks like you're going to let nature takes it's own course." He looked directly at me, and shaking his pointer finger, he declared, "Oh, no! If this gets to be a problem, I'm taking those pills!"

He died naturally the next day.

Tom had been appalled by the idea of dependency, but by having the ongoing love and respect of his wife and by still having choices, however narrow they became, his dignity remained intact. It was not dependency but fear of loss of value that frightened him the most. His family showed him he still had value. With love, care, and respect as a foundation, he had the strength to live out his days, even with the physical suffering that no one should be expected to tolerate. This is the dynamic I see again and again. I will not tell you it's easy, but remember, you have the hospice team to be your guides and your support.

> *The real work of dying means coming to terms with who you are, what the world is about, and what your place in it somehow is. It is a search for meaning.*
> —Dame Cecily Saunders, hospice founder

SECTION THREE

Communication—
Handle with Care

I'm Still Me

Who you are and who you've been doesn't change just because you now have a terminal prognosis. Do you like folk music? You still do. Do you chortle over risqué jokes told in whispered tones by that long-time buddy of yours? That probably won't change now, either. Do you love chocolate? The desire may or may not change, but the memory of your cravings won't. Are you the type who has been a bit cantankerous with a biting wit? Have you pushed away people in your past because you valued your independence above all else? You probably won't suddenly turn into Mr. Rogers.

The point here is that you are a fully-intact human being and will remain so until the moment of death, no matter how much your physical or mental abilities may change. As such, you are still allotted the full dimension of feelings, just like your family. Anger, guilt, joy, love, bitterness, humor, disappointment, frustration, and hopefulness—these feelings will always be a part of living.

There is sometimes the sense that when faced with a terminal illness, family especially must cherry pick only the pleasant, positive, and "acceptable" feelings. *Someone is dying, so we'd all better be on our best behavior. Let's not talk about the past or even the present if it's unpleasant.*

To express anger, frustration, or even humor is just not perceived as acceptable or respectful. We feel we must rise above our humanness and tap in only to our angelic selves and only see good in the person who is dying, no matter what the prior relationship has been. Within the belief that only the positive must be focused on now is the tendency to rewrite the past and deny, minimize, or trivialize our experiences. Have you ever been to the memorial service of someone you knew to be mean and selfish their whole life, and yet the deceased was described in flowery terms? You thought you were at the wrong service! That certainly wasn't describing the person you knew!

To edit and to censor some of our feelings and to deny our experiences is to deny our humanness. Does that mean it's OK to yell or list all the wrongs of a person? No, it means that you and your family have the right to retain your truths, to honor your feelings and your past, and to find the help you need to work through what may be painful issues. This may involve some tough conversations, but remember, hospice is there to help.

> *Some people weave burlap into the fabric of our lives, and some weave gold thread. Both contribute to make the whole picture beautiful and unique.*
> —Anonymous

Are you being seen and treated differently now? If you like it, great! If you discover you are missing your old patterns of communication, then speak up! Personally, I love to laugh. I would be upset if humor were considered taboo at my deathbed because that has been an important ingredient in my life. I want my family and friends to be telling their favorite funny stories so I can hear their laughter as I exit. Because I value humor, it is not only respectful to laugh at my deathbed, but it would be disrespectful *not* to, because this is who I am. Who are you, and what do you want? Talk about it with your loved ones, so in the end, you will all feel good that you left this earth in a way that honors who you are and they will feel good about their role in providing that.

To live in the hearts we leave behind is not to die.
—*Thomas Campbell*

Coulda, Woulda, Shoulda

Nobody can go back and start a new beginning,
but anyone can start today and make a new ending.
—Maria Robinson

What if the legacy you leave isn't one you are proud of? Is there forgiveness to be requested or forgiveness you need to offer? Does everyone you care about know how much they have meant to you? Are there regrets to be admitted or corrected? Now is not the time to judge your life and your choices—they were what they were. You have always been a human being with experiences, choices, and consequences for those choices, just like your family and friends. But if there are areas about which you feel you "coulda, woulda, or shoulda" done something different, it may not be too late to do something about it. After all, living or dying with regret is tough.

Here lies Jack Williams. He done his damndest.
Harry S. Truman asked to be remembered by this,
his favorite epitaph seen in Tombstone, Arizona.

I have witnessed much distress by those who hold on to anger, guilt, shame, and the like. It makes dying more difficult. Not everyone has had a great life or great relationships. There may be many hurts. There may be a painful history that seems insurmountable, and yet there is still the wish that all can be made better before death arrives. Cleaning up your life can be very freeing, but it's a challenge to suddenly learn a new skill or communicate in a new way. In this situation, getting the help of the hospice team will be of tremendous support to you and your family. Although it is common to hear that people often die the way they lived, there are also opportunities and possibilities at the end of life.

This can be a time of amazing personal transformations. Some people soften as they look toward the end of their lives, realizing finally that what was most important to them was their family and friends. They begin to appreciate the small kindnesses in ways never before felt. When faced with death, life can become excruciatingly beautiful in its short, fragile cycle. Sometimes the ability to give and receive love is the final lesson for those of us who have led lives distracted by achievements and external forces or who have taken for granted the love that has always been there for us.

It takes work and willingness on both parts to find healing. Although this healing is a positive thing, it doesn't always have to have a fairy-tale ending to be effective.

When Henry was admitted to the hospice inpatient unit, close to death, his one request was to speak to his daughter, Dolores. When called about his request for a visit, the daughter simply said, "No way!" Two more days passed, and even though circling death, Henry held on, requesting again and again to see his daughter. Another call was made, letting Dolores know of his urgent request, along with our belief that he was only holding onto life until this visit occurred. She grudgingly agreed to come in.

Dolores paused at the doorway, took a breath, and then proceeded to the bedside of her father. She looked down at the old man and declared, "You son of a bitch! You sexually molested me for the first fourteen years of my life. As a result, I've had three failed marriages, thirty years of counseling, I'll never have a normal relationship with a man, and I just hope you rot in hell!" She then turned and marched out the door, not wanting to wait for any response. After she walked out, Henry relaxed. The ugly truth had been spoken aloud, and within two hours, he died peacefully. In a sense, it freed Henry. Was it forgiveness? No. Some things will not be forgiven on this plane. It was the first and only time Dolores had faced her abuser. Giving her that time was Henry's only way to offer amends, as he knew there was no excuse for the actions of his past.

That confrontation would be another step toward his daughter's own healing work.

So healing and closure aren't always pretty, but they remain an important part of the work to be done by the patient, who needs to let go, and by the family, who needs to move forward.

Is transcendence of difficult histories also possible? Absolutely. I've been privileged to bear witness to forgiveness of old hurts, and to the ultimate giving and receiving of the love that had been withheld or rejected during life.

Claire

Claire always thought her father didn't love her and favored her older brother, who seemed to always get his attention. As much as she tried to gain his favor by getting good grades, helping at home, and succeeding in business, she still felt like she was never "seen" by him and never acknowledged for being a good and productive human being. This caused a lot of heartache. Her brother, on the other hand, seemed to get much in the way of personal counseling, support, and even financial help. Claire struggled with low self-esteem for thirty years, resenting her father's lack of attention, though still craving it at the same time. She never shared these feelings, fearing a final rejection.

Now her father was dying, and despite the pleas of her mother to "just say nice things," she could no longer hold it in. She confronted her father, told him of her pain and anger through the years, and asked why he didn't love her. Surprised at her outburst, he sat silently, and tears welled up in his eyes. Reaching for her hands, he said, "I'm so sorry, I thought you knew. You were so strong and beautiful and smart … I thought you didn't need me. Your brother was struggling, and I knew he needed help, but you … you always knew what to do, and I loved and admired you for that. I had no idea you thought I believed otherwise."

They hugged and cried together, creating the opening to talk about their lives, their successes, and their regrets, and achieve healing before his death one week later. Claire was so glad she took the risk to share her truths before he died.

Because your weeks or days are few, the healing of old wounds can be a fleeting yet wonderful gift for you, and an enduring and precious gift for those who live on.

You can't die cured, but you can die healed.
—*A hospice patient*

Final Wishes and Legacies

What still needs to be done before you leave this life? What dreams can still be achieved, but possibly in a modified form?

Ann

Ann had been looking forward to her trip to Hawaii after her retirement. She had planned this trip for three years, saving and waiting. One month prior to her retirement, she fell ill and was diagnosed with acute leukemia. She was not responding well to the treatments, and the chance of surviving looked slim. She returned home from the hospital with the support of hospice, working to reconcile the loss of her dream vacation. Knowing the pain of this loss, her friends and family got busy with planning. The following Saturday, they picked Ann up and took her to the home of a friend with a swimming pool. The patio had been decorated with tiki lights, palm fronds, and coconuts, everyone wore leis with hula skirts or Hawaiian shirts, and island music was playing. They hired a ukulele player to serenade Ann as they sipped on tropical drinks. They talked, laughed, and cried, and when the party was over, Ann thanked them profusely, stating this sharing with her friends and their acknowledgment of her dream was so much better than being alone in Hawaii. "You are all so much more beautiful than Hawaii," she said. "This has filled my soul, and I feel complete."

Hank

Hank loved being the life of the party. He cherished his friends and family as much as they did him. He jokingly stated he was going to miss not being at his own memorial service to hear the stories that would be told about him, and he wondered how he would be remembered. So a living memorial service was arranged—a party in which all friends and family were invited to share those stories that are usually saved for a traditional service after death. This way, the laughter and tears also brought validation, an acknowledgement of the impact Hank had on each person. Hank also designated time in which he could acknowledge each person in return. This simple sharing honored their relationships, focused on a life well lived (not just a life that was ending), and brought closure. The event was taped, and it continues to bring a smile to his wife, children, and grandchildren when they rerun the tapes and remember the man they loved and who loved them in return.

Chuck

Only thirty-four, Chuck was dying. His daughters were only four and six. He worried about how his wife would cope after his death and if his children would remember him, the love he had for them, and his dreams for each one. With the help of a hospice volunteer, he videotaped messages to his family with the directions that the tape was to be viewed only after his death. Years later, this family reports that whenever they are feeling down or facing difficult times, they look at this tape to feel strengthened by his love.

Think about the memories you want to leave. Do you want time alone with each person, or do you want to write or dictate final messages? What about the environment in which you want to spend your final days? Tell your loved ones if you want special music, readings, or silence in your final hours. Do you want your bed facing an open window to feel the breeze and hear the birds feeding outside? Your loved ones will be grateful to know your wishes and to be able to fulfill them. This is the time for everyone to ask for what they need.

The only thing you take with you when you're gone is
what you leave behind.
—*John Allston*

The Need for Intimacy

Intimacy—the ability to be fully who you are with someone, physically,
emotionally, and/or spiritually; to see and be fully seen and still be loved
and cherished.

Because we are fully intact human beings until our last breath, our need for intimacy and human connectedness does not change. Physically, emotionally, and spiritually, the need may even increase as we face our final months and days on earth.

Human touch is a very potent elixir. We know it increases our natural endorphins, our internal morphine, which enhances a sense of well-being and even strengthens our immune system. Yet as people become sicker and more frail, the tendency is to touch less—usually for fear of hurting that person, being seen as selfish, or just behaving inappropriately when someone is near the end of life.

A Tale of Two Taboos

Only the topic of death is more taboo than the topic of sexuality. Combine the two, and you've got something that very few people are comfortable talking about. This human need is often swept under the bed rather than its place acknowledged on top of it. Even hospice, for all its purported focus on mind, body, spirit, patient, and family, fails to include barriers to intimacy on the list of care plan options to be addressed. Our sexuality and our humanness will always be a part of who we are.

Yes, decreasing energy and sexual desire may be a part of the overall physical decline, and sex may be the least of your interests. But this will vary with people at different times in their illness. Don't be afraid to express your needs or desires. For the men, are there medications that may affect your ability to achieve an erection? If so, don't take them prior to lovemaking. Is pain a part of your disease process? If so, how long before should you take your medication to assure comfort? Are there positions that will allow you to expend less energy and enjoy the contact more? Do you need to take your breathing meds just beforehand, and should you increase your oxygen? What are the barriers that need to be addressed? Do you need to empty the colostomy bag or fold back the catheter? And why don't medical-supply companies make double-sized hospital beds? These are all questions you should be able to ask your physician or hospice team.

Sex is not the only choice in intimacy, just the one we consider least in terminal illness. Hugging each other, spooning, holding hands, talking about the highlights of your life together, enjoying a simple massage, falling asleep in each other's arms, brushing hair, kissing fingers and noses, laughing, crying … they are all just types of intimacy. If intimacy is still important to you or if you feel like less of a man or woman because it has been excluded from your day-to-day existence, say something. Some of these gestures of intimacy are not just for your spouse or life partner, but also for your children, your parents, and your friends. It's one way we connect with each other.

You're Going to Miss Me, Right?— Opening The Door To Communicating What Is Important

Many of us have learned that when faced with a painful situation, the best course is to not show our feelings. Suck it up. Hold it in. Pretend we are strong and nothing will affect us. If this is your way, how can you and your family effectively find closure? Your heart is breaking, but you hold back the tears. There is often a silent conspiracy to try not to talk about what's happening, because it might break that fragile facade. What's the worst that can happen? You may cry together. Your humanness and connectedness will be revealed to each other. What's so bad about that?

Andy was a man who was adored by everyone who knew him. Bedridden, his friends and family would take turns visiting at his bedside, sharing stories, and laughing, like the good old days. When they left his room, however, they would fall into each other's arms in tears, devastated by the fact that they would soon lose their beloved friend and family member. During a routine hospice visit, Andy confided in his hospice nurse that he was angry and hurt. When asked about the reason, he pointed to the many pictures of friends and family on his wall and dresser and exclaimed, "No one even cares that I'm dying! Do you know that no one has even shed a tear?"

It was time for the grief to come out of the back room to be shared by all.

In sharing our sadness and our grief, we share our hearts and our love. The cost of loving someone is that it will hurt like a son-of-a-gun when they die. Holding in our sadness is much more painful than sharing it. The only way to prevent this pain is to never love in the first place, and how would that affect our quality of life?

The only feelings that do not heal are the ones you hide.

—Henry Nouwen

I encourage you and your loved ones to open up, to share memories, to talk about what you each will miss most after you are gone, and to talk about what you have learned from each other. Will this bring tears? Very often, yes. Is this a bad thing? No. It will be more painful if you die without ever telling your loved ones what they meant to you or if you die without ever being told what you mean to them. That's when grief becomes complicated and more painful than it already is. Can't start with the words? Write a letter. Hand it to the person while you are with him or her. Sit in silence while he/she reads it. Things will unfold from there. This simple communication lets each of you know your shared lives had meaning. How different would our lives be if we didn't wait until death to let people know how we feel? Then sudden deaths wouldn't be as painful as they are when things are left unsaid.

The bitterest tears shed over graves are for
words left unsaid and deeds left undone
—Harriet Beecher Stow

Children Matter

Children, grandchildren, that adorable five-year-old neighbor who has adopted you as surrogate parent ... if they have been a part of your life, they will be affected by your dying. Children pick up signs of distress from others, and that can increase their own fears or even their sense of guilt if they are not a part of what is happening. Talk with the hospice social worker or bereavement counselor about how best to deal with children, because there will be differences depending on their ages and maturity. There are also wonderful books available that an adult can read with the child to enhance understanding and promote a sense of acceptance and peace. The nice thing is that when we do this for the children, it comforts us as well.

Children may express their fear and grief by acting out, withdrawing, creating a fantasy world, and more, depending on their age and the responses of the adults around them. They can even create a belief that they are somehow responsible for the death, which can haunt them for many years. The hospice team can assist you in communicating with and understanding children during this time and in bereavement. Like you, they will benefit from caring assistance.

Just like adults, a child can feel a sense of helplessness. To promote a sense that they are helping you, suggest an age-appropriate task they can complete:

"I'd love for you to draw me one of your special pictures. I want to put it right here where I can see it."

"Can you read me your favorite story?"

"Sing to me."

"Rub lotion on my hand. That feels so much better. Thank you so much for helping me!"

That little person will remember making a positive difference. Tell the child what you love about him/her. Ask the child what he/she will remember about you, and be prepared for smiles and laughter with the answers!

Don't Forget the Four-Footed

Your dog, your cat, or even your bird may also be affected by your dying, so don't forget to include them. Animals are more accepting of death than we humans. Your pet may choose to stay close by, giving and receiving comfort. Some may also opt to watch only from a distance, or detach completely, because they sense what is happening and don't struggle with the human challenge of letting go.

If you die in the hospital, ask your family to leave an article of your clothing near the pet's bedding to provide comfort. If you are on the inpatient hospice unit, remember that pets are welcomed and even encouraged to visit. After death, ask your family to give pets the opportunity to see your body and to help them understand the person they knew no longer resides there. That diminishes a possible sense of abandonment.

Pets can also grieve and need comforting. Ask your family to watch for changes in behavior, like not eating or playing, and talk to the vet if their health seems at risk.

Details, Details

As you and your family prepare for death, you must also prepare for what happens after death. Makings plans for a funeral or cremation may include where, how, in what dress, and in what time frame. If there is a service, is there a special reading or music you want provided? If you are to be buried, are there religious or financial restrictions regarding the coffin? What about embalming or cremation? These details are good to handle early on, so you can participate, if you so desire. You'll want to make sure your wishes are followed and that your family doesn't have to wonder or argue among themselves about whether they are doing the right thing by you.

The paperwork necessary after a death is sometimes overwhelming. You will need to let your family know where important papers and accounts are kept, if they don't already know. This can include documentation about military service, retirement accounts, lock box keys, custody issues, your marriage certificate, titles, pet placement, stock options, your last will and testament, and the like. Searching for these papers after a death adds needless stress and strain on a family that is already mourning. It is a gift from you to handle this ahead of time with them.

Some people don't want to handle this early on for fear of being jinxed—that if they are prepared ahead of time, death might take them ahead of time. Others fear what their family might do with this information. Still others never want to admit that the end is near and by not talking about these things, the reality doesn't have to be acknowledged.

In the letting-go process, people often want to know their loved ones will be OK without them. You want to know they have the skills, support, and information they need to move forward in their lives. If you are worried about them, it may be more difficult for you to let go, so beginning the dialogue about these final arrangements is very important. Because of the emotions that may be involved, the hospice team can help you so everyone is heard and all issues are handled as best as possible.

What If I Wake Up Dead?

Let's state the obvious first. If you are dead, you will no longer be waking up—at least not here.

But some people carry the fear that they won't really be dead, but that they will wake up in a morgue and be unable to communicate their predicament prior to being embalmed or incinerated. Indeed, this is a thought that taps into our deepest fears, those that assure the success of horror movies. Some of this comes from many years ago, before there were stethoscopes to listen to and determine when the heart and lungs stopped working. Occasionally, people were in deep stupors or comas and suddenly awoke, finding themselves buried in their coffins. To avoid this problem, a string was attached to the dead person's wrists, brought through the coffin to the area above the grave, and attached to a bell. That way, if he woke up, the bell would be rung, and the ever-alert cemetery worker on duty, who had been specifically listening for any ringing, would respond by digging up that person immediately. Thus, the term "dead ringer" was born.

There have been many advances that preclude the need for that now, yet the fear and the rare stories remain. Although I hope my assurances here will calm you, if this is your fear, share it with your family. Ask your funeral home what their checks and balances are to make sure you are dead. What I can tell you is that at the time of death, there is a definite sense that the person is gone—that the spirit no longer inhabits the body, which is now an empty shell. There is no life when circulation and breathing have stopped. Consciousness ceases, and all feeling is gone.

You may want to attend a group meeting for those who have had a near-death experience or read one of the many books and articles on this phenomena. They can provide a glimpse into the mystery of dying and about what happens at the moment of death—how your spirit leaves your body and discovers peace and joy and is not left behind to decay with your physical body. When a group member exclaims, "I can hardly wait to die again!" well, how bad can it be? Again and again, people describe a sense of peace. All pain and fear is gone and is replaced by a knowing that all is well. As I have watched many deaths, I also see and feel a profound sense of peace.

We have ways of covering up death and sanitizing it, which can contribute to us not seeing its reality. If you have only seen a dead person who has been made up by the mortician and looks "lifelike," like they may just sit up and yawn after an extended nap, remember that the makeup provides a surreal illusion. It's what the person looks like before the makeup that is real.

For those who have experienced the "visitation" of a person who has died (this may be more common than you think), there has never been talk from the deceased about suffering after death or feeling cremation or embalming. Consistently, the talk is of achieving profound peace and joy regarding their final release. There are many books about this, which you may find comforting to read.

So you will not "wake up dead" in this world, though you may wake up "alive" in the next one.

Death is simply a shedding of the physical body like the butterfly
shedding its cocoon. It is a transition to a higher state of
consciousness where you continue to perceive, to understand,
to laugh, and to be able to grow.
—Elizabeth Kubler Ross

SECTION FOUR

The Mystery

The Timing of Death

The most beautiful thing we can experience is the mysterious.
—Albert Einstein

Talking about the timing of death is entering into an exploration of one of the mysteries of dying. While this section may be more useful to your loved ones, given your decreasing level of consciousness and your increased willingness to let go, reading it may help open you to further appreciate the mystery of dying.

I've had many patients tell me when they were going to die—sometimes to the day and sometimes to the minute. This inner knowing isn't always something that you can consciously be aware of and share with your family. But have faith that everything will happen exactly as it is supposed to. Now let me explain what I mean by that.

What I and so many hospice and end-of-life workers have come to know is that there is an enigma around the timing of death. The time is set. I let families know ahead of time that if they are supposed to be there at the time of your death, they will be, and if they are not supposed to be there, they won't be. There is no judgment about either possibility. It doesn't mean someone is good because they were there or bad because they just left when it happened. Too many people hold onto guilt for years after a death. They make statements such as, "I just walked out of the room to get coffee," or "I took too long to get dressed before I came back to visit." For reasons we may never know on this plane, that person simply wasn't supposed to be with the dying person at the time of death. Again and again, I have seen patients in the hospital die during shift changes, when no one was around to disturb them. I've also seen patients die just before or just after someone visited, and I've seen those who waited for the arrival of a certain person or a special day.

> *Alicia was declining quickly from her breast cancer, which had spread to other key organs in her body. Her wish was to know her son, fighting the war in Iraq, was safe. After many phone calls and letters, the military released her son to visit the bedside of his dying mother. He called from the airport the moment his plane landed, and within one minute of receiving that call, his mother died. The son was distraught that he arrived too late, but as the family talked about the timing of this death, it was felt she just wanted to make sure her son arrived safely, and to spare him the pain of seeing her final breath. The son acknowledged he would have had a difficult time seeing that. With this timing of her death, the son was assured that his first and final view was of his mother in peaceful repose in her bed, a contented look on her face that remained even in death.*

Sometimes the timing is about a last wish ...

> *When Helen was admitted to the hospice inpatient unit from the intensive care unit, she expressed a final wish—to be divorced before her death. Apparently, when she became seriously ill, her husband left her and soon moved in with a younger woman. Helen*

wanted the divorce finalized to assure her assets would go directly to her daughter, not to her husband. The final hearing was to be the coming Monday at 1 pm. She just needed to stay alive until just after 1 pm on Monday to achieve her final wish of a divorce.

Over the weekend, Helen lapsed into a coma, and the hospice staff grew nervous. 1 PM on Monday—that's all she needed to reach to realize her wish. However, Helen continued to decline. Monday arrived, and at 11:05, Helen died. We were devastated that she had gotten so close, yet didn't get her wish. We called her daughter to report her death and our own agony of Helen not getting that final wish. The daughter asked, "What do you mean?" We replied, "The divorce hearing that was supposed to be at 1. She died before she could be divorced." The daughter softly responded, "I didn't tell you. I got the hearing moved up to 11."

Sometimes it's about being released ...

Donald's family adored him. They were devastated that he was dying, and they were committed to his not dying alone. Seventeen family members participated in a deathwatch, making sure he was never alone. They were also having a hard time letting go, and each time Donald drifted off to sleep, they would grab his arm and exclaim, "Dad! Dad! Stay with us! We love you!" Donald was never allowed to relax or do the work of dying (see the chapter You Just Gonna Sleep?). The family, in terrible grief, could not find the strength to let him go.

On the third day of the vigil, an exhausted Donald whispered weakly into the ear of his nurse, "Get them out of here!" The nurse and social worker requested that the family meet with them in a quiet room to handle mortuary arrangements. Within two minutes of them leaving, Donald died. He needed his release. The family was upset with us, but we didn't tell them what Donald had said so as not to complicate their grief with a feeling of guilt. But this emphasizes the need for letting go, closure, and the role of timing.

So I tell families ahead of time that the timing of death is already determined. They may ask, "We've been here since 6 AM and need to get something to eat ... do you think we have time to go to a fast food place?" My answer is, "I don't know. Tell your loved one you are leaving and when you will return, whether he's in a coma or not (remember what I told you about hearing). If he wants to wait for you, he will. If he wants to die while you are gone, he will. Let it go. It will be done his way, and hopefully you can find comfort in knowing that."

Succumbing to the mystery and timing of death is a process for patient and family alike.

Dreams, Visions, and Messages

Seeing death as the end of life is like seeing
the horizon as the end of the ocean.
—David Searls

Dying is as much a mystery as being born. We all have our own beliefs about death and whether or not there is life after death. There is so much we simply won't know until we get there. But those getting closer to the end of their lives seem to have an expanded awareness, and often images and information arrive in different ways. Are you having unusual dreams? Do you find yourself talking to relatives who have already died? Are you watching glimpses of your past? Are you arguing with someone about wanting to go or wanting to stay?

Do not be alarmed if this is happening, as it is a very common occurrence. Although no one else can see or hear what you do, it doesn't mean it isn't real and that you must discredit what you see. It's very real to you, and there are often important messages within these visions, which may be received from dead relatives, friends, animals, children, or religious figures.

Visions are not just deathbed occurrences and may occur days or even months prior to death. Why we are more open to receiving these visions near the end of life, I don't know. Perhaps it's a part of letting go of pretense and of opening ourselves up more to the universe, or maybe it's a willingness and desire to experience the mystery and sacredness of living and dying.

Many patients tell me their sense of reality begins to blur and that they have difficulty telling the difference between being asleep and being awake. Some have described it as being between two worlds and need reorientation when awakened. Your family may hear you using symbolic speech, reflecting your level of readiness to let go of life. Common phrases include, "I want to go home!" "I don't want to go yet!" "Where are the keys?" "I need my ticket,"

"Where's the bus?" "I need to pack my suitcase," and "Where is my wedding dress?" (The last statement was from a woman close to death who looked forward to rejoining her husband, who had died years before.) While your awareness at this time is usually such that you are barely or no longer able to carry on a real conversation with your loved ones, those who surround you have the opportunity to glimpse another reality through you.

Harriet

Harriet was a fiercely-independent woman in her seventies. Having kicked out her husband years before, she raised her two children by herself. She had disliked the interference of her family, but had enjoyed the company of a few friends. At the time she entered the hospice program, both her family and friends had died and her two children were estranged from each other and had only limited contact with Harriet.

She had no belief in any religious dogma or afterlife, declaring, "When you're dead, you're dead. That's it!" Her daughter, on the other hand, had aspired to become a nun, but due to some unfortunate politics, was unable to complete this training, thus causing her to experience her own faith crisis. While Harriet was not interested in talking about dying and the possibility of visions, her daughter was.

Preferring her privacy, Harriet's desire was to die quickly at home so no one had the chance to take her anywhere or fuss over her. She got her wish. On a Thursday visit, I found her to be declining rapidly. I got her into bed and called her daughter. We sat on either side of Harriet's bed as she slipped into a semicomatose state. What was unusual was that she essentially talked through her dying.

"Where's the bus? The bus is late!" she'd angrily declare from her reclining position with her eyes closed. Now I understood this metaphor about the bus, but wasn't sure how to respond, since I was a relatively new hospice nurse. I finally decided to offer a

comforting statement. "The bus will be coming." Feeling braver, I added, "… and family will be there to help you." Still semicomatose, she grimaced and sarcastically responded, "Oh goody!" I had forgotten how she disliked her family.

The ranting continued. "Where's the bus? The bus is late!" she proclaimed. Finally, she reported that a bus had shown up, and we presumed she would get on it. After a few minutes of silence, she declared, "I can't stay on this bus—this is the bus to hell!" Taken aback and not knowing what to say, I offered, "Get off the bus!" This is when I first discovered what seems to be a universal law—that if you have a vision you don't like, you can ask it to go away, and it will. Nobody can ask for you. You alone provide that direction. So Harriet "got off the bus to hell," and the ranting began again. "Where's the bus? The bus is late!" she exclaimed.

After many minutes, she reported that a white ambulance showed up, and I asked if that was OK. "Yes," she responded gruffly. All was quiet for several more minutes, and then suddenly, the energy in the room changed. Though still semicomatose, Harriet's body literally lit up with joy as her hands raised to her face, and she exclaimed, "Look! It's a party! And they've been waiting for me all this time!" She was grinning ear to ear, and lord knows I had never seen this woman even crack a smile in the last four months. She was literally beaming with joy while she happily reported that it was her friends at the party, not family. The daughter, still sitting across from me with tears streaming down her face, said, "I know you told me this was possible, but until this moment, I couldn't believe it."

How wonderful that in sharing her dying experience, a woman with no belief system reaffirmed the faith of her daughter and offered me a glimpse into the mystery of dying. She "partied it up" for another three hours until she drew her last breath and joined her friends.

Jeremy

Only twenty-seven, Jeremy lay close to death, surrounded by his family and his hospice nurse. Still able to talk, he pointed to the end of his bed and asked, "Who is that little boy?" When nobody could respond because they didn't see any boy, Jeremy described him—he had blond hair and blue eyes, and he was about three. His mother gasped and hurried out of the room. Moments later, she returned with a small picture of a three-year-old blond-haired boy. Looking at the picture, Jeremy stated, "Yes, that's him! How did you get his picture?" His mother had never told him he had a brother who had died at the age of three, before Jeremy was born. Now, in the midst of the pain of losing a second son, his mother had a modicum of comfort in knowing that her two sons were soon to be together and that now there was the possibility she would see them both again one day.

As you share your experiences, you have the opportunity to expand the awareness of the awesomeness of this amazing time with those who love you. It will never take away the pain of the loss, but it can introduce them to the mystery and help them face future deaths with less fear and greater awareness.

My Wish for You

I wish you strength. May there be healing where it is needed. May your wishes be fulfilled. May you and your loved ones touch the extraordinary, realize the possibilities, and experience the mystery. May you live your days in comfort, love, and peace.

I honor your life and your journey.

There are only two ways to live your life.
One is as though nothing is a miracle.
The other is as if everything is.
—Albert Einstein

Parting Words

"It's very beautiful over there."
—Last words of Thomas Edison

"Why should I talk to you? I've just been talking to your boss."
—Wilson Mizner, US writer, gained consciousness briefly while
on his deathbed and discovered a priest standing over him

"Either the wallpaper goes, or I do."
—Last words of Oscar Wilde

"Now comes the mystery ..."
—Last words of Henry Ward Beecher

*Curtain! Fast music! Lights! Ready for the last finale! Great.
The show looks good, the show looks good!*
—Last words of Florenz Ziegfeld, producer of the renowned
Ziegfeld Follies, a dance troupe of the early 1900s

Aftermath for the Survivors

Self-Care First

If you haven't been to your doctor because of all the attention you've given to your loved one, now is the time. The physical and emotional work you have done can take a toll on your body, and this is a good first step to begin to take care of yourself again. Have you lost touch with good friends because you've been too busy? Call them up, go to lunch, or take a walk together. Have you missed your weekly tennis, yoga, dancing, or art classes? Rejoin them. You will benefit from reconnecting with the world that you once enjoyed. This is the time that must be about *you*.

Grief—It Just Hurts

Grief is not limited to the time after death. Grief can happen as soon as loss is anticipated. Grief can happen with each physical loss and with each change in a relationship. There's also the anticipatory grief of knowing someone you love will die. You've already experienced this. Now there's a whole new level of grief compounded by the fact there will be no more memories to make together. There is nobody to reminisce about the past that you both shared. There is nobody for whom you can provide medications, back rubs, or sips of water at three in the morning. The person you centered your life around while providing care is now gone, and you are out of that job, as well as a shared life.

Your whole being will react to this loss.

Physically you may experience:
- shakiness or edginess;
- headaches;
- chest or throat pain or tightness;
- stomach hollowness;
- lack of energy;
- the same symptoms as the deceased;
- hunger or loss of appetite;
- dry mouth;
- nausea;
- extra sensitivity to noise.

Emotionally you may experience:
- sadness;
- shock;
- guilt;
- fear;
- relief;
- numbness;

- anger or irritation;
- frustration;
- helplessness;
- lack of control;
- longing;
- dread;
- Disbelief;
- preoccupation with the deceased.

Behaviors may include:
- eating too much or too little;
- increased use of alcohol, drugs, or nicotine;
- sleeping too much or too little;
- searching behavior—expecting the deceased;
- increase or decrease in activity;
- absent-mindedness;
- change in work performance;
- crying;
- visiting or avoiding places that remind you of the deceased.

You may feel like you are going crazy or that there is something seriously wrong with you, but all of the above are *normal* reactions to grief.

Bereavement Groups

I seem to be falling apart.
My attention span can be measured in seconds.
My patience in minutes.
I cry at the drop of a hat.
I forget to sign the checks.
Half of everything in the house is misplaced.
Feelings of anxiety and restlessness are my constant companions.
Rainy days seem extra dreary.
Sunny days seem an outrage.
Other people's pain and frustration seem insignificant.
Laughing, happy people seem out of place in my world.
It has become routine to feel half crazy.
I am normal I am told.
I am a newly grieving person.
—Anonymous

Danger Signs

If you are experiencing suicidal thoughts, if you are unable to manage your daily needs, such as bathing, shopping, eating, and taking care of your own health, or if you are using drugs or alcohol to numb the pain, then you need to seek the help of a professional right away. You may not have the emotional energy to make this call, so please let a family member or friend know so help can be found.

I Thought I'd Feel Better by Now

- *It's been seven months, and I cry at the drop of a hat. I can't concentrate, and I'm irritable. There must be something wrong with me!*
- *I can't cry—I'm too angry. How could he have left me? Why didn't he fight to live?*
- *My family is sick of my tears and wanting to talk about my son. They think I should just move on.*
- *I have so many regrets. What can I do about them now?*
- *He was such a horrid father. He hurt me, and I hated him for that. I thought I'd feel better now that he's gone.*
- *It's been six weeks, and I don't feel back to normal. I should be feeling better by now, shouldn't I?*

First of all, as one wise man told me, *"Don't 'should' on yourself!"*

As you can see from the above statements that I've heard from bereaved families and friends, the grief experience is different for each person. The work of grief is also different for each person. It's a lifelong process, and everyone has a different way of proceeding. Just know that you do not need to feel alone on this journey. It's a sad irony that the one event we will all share as human beings—losing someone or something we love—is also an event that tends to makes us feel very alone, as though nobody else could ever understand the meaning of our loss or the depth of our pain. This is not the time to isolate yourself, but to explore the meaning of grief for you and how to best work through it.

First the bad news—the grief process is probably a lot harder and longer than you ever thought possible. The full impact of your loss may not happen for days, months, or sometimes even years after a death. You may also experience more pain around a birthday, anniversary, or other special occasion that you used to share with the deceased. There will be days of intolerable pain and also days when you smile with memories and feel "almost normal." There will be no avoiding it—the grief process is a roller coaster, and you're going to want good "grab bars" to help you hold on.

Now the good news—there are people who can help and who can be your "grab bars." Your hospice bereavement counselor or a grief support group is a good place to start. It is not a sign of weakness that you need support, but rather a sign of strength that you can reach out and begin the hard work of grieving. Most of us have not been taught these skills, and even when we have, it doesn't make it easier. Give yourself permission to find the support and comfort you deserve.

Where there is sorrow there is holy ground.
—Oscar Wilde

Coping Well—What Does That Even Mean?

Your father has died, and your brother seems to be handling it well. He reminisces with a smile, is involved in his work, and is talking about taking a vacation. But you can't talk without crying, can't concentrate at work, and can't imagine making plans without including your father. Does that mean he is coping and you aren't? Or is he "doing it wrong" by not outwardly grieving like you are? The answer is absolutely not on both counts.

Everyone has his or her own way. Some are expressive in their grief, while others say nothing. Some want a ceremony with all involved, while others only deal with it in private. Some seem to get busier than ever, while others withdraw from activity. Some want to get rid of everything that reminds them of the person who died, while others create an untouchable shrine in the room the deceased used to occupy. Find someone with whom you can share your grief in the way that is natural for you. If it irritates you to be with a person who has a different way of coping, then avoid that person for now. Don't judge or allow yourself to be judged for the way that is comfortable for you.

Now What?

I am not a grief counselor, and I admit to simplifying the grieving process above, providing only the tip of the proverbial iceberg about grief. Just like I introduced this book to let you know you are not alone in the dying process, I would like to inform you that you need not be alone in the grieving process. And just like your loved one was encouraged to reach out and accept help prior to death, you are encouraged to do the same. I strongly encourage you to seek grief counselors or groups, read one of the many insightful and helpful books on grief, or go online. Finding a trusted friend or family member who will sit with you as you recount your experiences again and again is also very healing.

Allow people to help you, and you will all benefit. You will never forget the one who died. That person will forever be a part of your heart and your life. Honor those memories and honor yourself by continuing your own life's journey.

We must embrace the pain
and burn it to fuel our journey.
—Kenji Miyazawa

A Death Has Occurred

A death has occurred and everything is changed.
We are painfully aware
that life can never be the same again,
that yesterday is over,
that relationships once rich have ended.
But there is another way to look upon this truth.
If life now went on the same,
without the presence of the one who has died,
we could only conclude that the life we remember
made no contribution, filled no space, meant nothing.
The fact that this person left behind a place
that cannot be filled
is a high tribute to this individual.
Life can be the same after a trinket has been lost,
but never after the loss of a treasure.
—Paul Iron

Resources

CDs

Graceful Passages: A Companion for Living and Dying. Published by New World Library. *Produced by Michael Stillwater and Gary Malkin for Wisdom of the World Productions. Www.wisdomoftheworld.com.* Unspeakable Grace: The Music of Graceful Passages *Music Composed by Gary Malkin.* Produced by Wisdom of the World. Www.wisdomoftheworld.com.

Recommended Readings

Ablom, Mitch, *Tuesdays With Morrie.*

Byock, Ira, *Dying Well: The Prospect for Growth at the End of Life.*

Callahan, M and Kelley, P, *Final Gifts.*

Levine, Stephen, *A Year to Live.*

Lynne MD, Joanne, *Handbook for Mortals—Guidance for People Facing Serious Illness.*

Singh, Kathleen Dowling, *The Grace in Dying.*

Wolfelt, Alan, *The Journey Through Grief: Reflections on Healing.*

Wolfelt, Alan, *Understanding Your Grief: Ten Essential Touchstones for Finding Hope and Healing Your Heart.*

Bibliography

Arnold, R., "Fast Facts and Concepts #83: Why Patients Do Not Take Their Opioids," February 2003, End-of-Life Physician Resource Center, www.eperc.mcw.edu.

"Artificial Nutrition and Hydration at the End of Life," 2006, Caring Connections, National Hospice and Palliative Care Organization.

Callahan Pflaum, Maggie and Kelley, Patricia, "Understanding the Final Messages of the Dying," *Nursing 86*, June.

Counseling Your Patients and Their Families Regarding the Use of Opioids to Relieve Pain, 2000, Partners against Pain, Purdue Pharma L.P.

Cross, Karen, "If He Would Just Eat, I Know He Would Get Stronger: Eating and Drinking at the End of Life," *Quarterly Newsletter of the American Academy of Hospice and Palliative Medicine*, Fall 2001.

"Dispel Misconceptions About Morphine," American Academy of Hospice and Palliative Medicine.

Dunn, Hank, *Hard Choices for Loving People*.

Fainsinger, Robin, "Fast Facts and Concept #133: Non-Oral Hydration in Palliative Care,"

End-of-Life Physician Resource Center, www.eperc.mcs.edu.

Finucane, T.E., Christmas, C., Travis, K., "Tube Feeding in Patients with Advanced Dementia." JAMA. 1999; 282:1365-1369.

Hallenbeck, J., Weissman, D., "Fast Fact and Concept #10: Tube Fed or Not Tube Feed?"

End-of-Life Physician Resource Center, www.eperc.mcw.edu.

Marchand, Lucille, "Fast Fact and Concept #118: Near Death Awareness," End-of-Life Physician Resource Center, www. eperc.mcw.edu.

Morris, Virginia, *Talking About Death Won't Kill You*.

Rousseau, Paul, "How Fluid Deprivation Affects the Terminally Ill."

Weisman, D., "Fast Facts and Concepts #08: Morphine and Hastened Death," June 2000. End-of-Life Physician Resource Center, www.eperc.mcw.edu.

Worden, J. William, *Grief Counseling and Grief Therapy*, 1992.

Internet Resources

These are only a few of the many websites with valuable information about end-of-life issues. You can search for hospice, death and dying, grief and loss, bereavement, or end of life and find numerous additional resources online.

www.NHPCO.com

www.hospicefoundation.org

www.hospicenet.org

www.aarp.org

www.eperc.mcw.edu

www.care-giver.com

www.griefloss.org

www.grieflossrecovery.com